KETOGENIC DIET

A Quick, No B.S. Guide to Rapid Fat Loss

Table of Contents

Introduction

As more and more people are becoming obese, an endless supply of so-called diets are popping up left, right and center offering solutions. The problem is many of them aren't legit as many of them were just concocted in the dark, stuffy confines of pseudo-dieticians' minds and were released to the world via the Internet, where it's hard to distinguish between what's legit and what isn't.

Fortunately, many bad apples don't spoil the whole bunch and there are still good diets that are – well – legit! And one of those is the ketogenic diet. It's legit because thousands of people and many scientific studies have already verified its legitimacy as an effective weight loss diet – with other benefits to boot! And in this book, you'll learn about the ketogenic diet, why it's the best, and how to use it to your advantage. Plus, you'll also learn a few easy and delicious recipes to help you to stick to it, as how to stay on the diet while eating out.

So what are you waiting for? Turn the page and let's begin!

CHAPTER 1: Ketogenic Diet 101

The ketogenic diet is one that features low carbohydrate intake with a high dietary fat intake. While it may seem unhealthy, given the relatively higher fat content, it's a diet that offers many benefits to your health. There have been many studies that have already shown that the ketogenic diet not only helps people lose weight, but also achieve much better health.

You may be wondering what the story is behind the name of the diet. The word ketogenic, often called keto, is derived from the word ketosis. It is a metabolic state where your body can become a very effective fat burning machine as a means of generating energy.

Greatly reducing the intake or consumption of carbohydrates and significantly increasing the consumption or intake of dietary fat achieve ketosis. Also, this process helps your body transform body fat into a substance called ketone inside the liver. Ketones are an excellent supply or source of energy for your brain. Many who have gone through this diet attest to experiencing significant improvements in their mental performance as well as substantial reductions, if not elimination, of a mental condition referred to as brain fog.

Ketogenic Diet Types

There are several different types of ketogenic diets, but these can be generally grouped into four types:

The standard ketogenic diet (SKD), high protein ketogenic diet, the targeted ketogenic diet (TKD), and the cyclical ketogenic diet (CKD).

The standard ketogenic diet is one that only has 5% carbohydrates, 20% protein, and a whopping 75% made up of dietary fat. The targeted ketogenic diet is a version of the standard ketogenic diet that allows for additional carbohydrates to be consumed immediately before and after exercising or working out.

The cyclical ketogenic diet is one where you go on the standard ketogenic diet for 5 straight days followed by two days with high carbohydrate consumption. Lastly, the high protein ketogenic diet is the higher protein version of the standard one, where dietary fat drops to only 60% of total calories and protein increases to 35% of total daily calories.

But in terms of scientific study backing, only the standard and the high protein ketogenic diets were subjected to extensive scientific studies. This is because elite athletes and bodybuilders, both of which comprised only a very small segment of the population, mostly use the two other versions, the targeted and the cyclical versions. For the purposes of reading this book, keep in mind that we will be focusing on the standard ketogenic diet. While that may be the case, many principles surrounding the standard diet can also be applied to the three other versions.

CHAPTER 2: Ketogenic Diet and Weight Loss

The single largest reason why the ketogenic diet is very popular all over the world is weight loss. Let's admit it – seldom do people go on a "diet" for health reasons alone. Most of the time, it is merely aesthetic. There's no shame in that – looking good and feeling fit is truly important for one's sense of self-esteem.

But the truth is, even the seemingly shallow vanity reason for weight loss isn't as vain as you may think it is. This is because being overweight – obese being the more scientific term – and suffering other related metabolic diseases has grown into epidemic proportions in the last 20 years or so. Think of it this way:

- Every year, almost 3 million adults die as a result of causes related to obesity; and

- In the United States alone, more than 50 million people are at risk of a wide range of health problems due to being afflicted with a medical condition known as metabolic syndrome.

As a result of the increasing health risks due to the increasing incidence of obesity and metabolic diseases, many "diets" have popped up in an attempt to address the problem. These are meant to help people lose weight and most of them promise to lead to really fast weight loss. Many of these diets, however, aren't backed up by reputable scientific studies and, as such, a certain number of these diets aren't healthy or realistic. In fact, many of them tend to be too restrictive and lead to a boomerang or rubber band effect, where the dieters eventually gain back their original weight and then some.

The ketogenic diet, fortunately for us, is backed up by scientific studies to be both effective and healthy.

The Science behind the Weight Loss

As mentioned earlier, a ketogenic diet is one that's loaded with dietary fat, has moderate amounts of protein and very few carbohydrates, if at all, which brings the body into a metabolic state known as ketosis – the root word from which the diet got its name. The weight loss from this type of diet is the real weight loss you and I need to experience – fat loss. Much weight loss provided by other diets involves a great deal of water and muscle mass and when you lose significant muscle mass, your metabolism slows down. That's the reason why so many people plateau in their weight loss endeavors after only a week or two even if they severely restrict their calories – a great deal of muscle mass loss is involved rather than fat loss.

When your body's in a state of ketosis for a prolonged period of time, it learns to tap into body fat for energy instead of carbohydrates, which leads to more fat loss than muscle mass loss when it comes to weight loss.

As mentioned earlier, the ketogenic diet is backed up by scientific studies when it comes to losing weight – the right kind of weight. Compared to most other diets out there, it can help you preserve or even build muscle mass while losing body fat. And this is on top of many health improvements, which we'll discuss in another chapter.

One of the most popular diets aimed at promoting healthy weight or fat loss is the low fat diet. And when the ketogenic diet – a high fat diet – is compared to low fat diets, many scientific studies vouch for the ketogenic diet over low fat diets. In particular, these studies have shown the ketogenic diet to be superior even if total caloric intake's the same. In one study, the ketogenic diet resulted in an average weight loss of more than twice that of a low fat and low calorie diet. More than that, the same study also showed improvements in HDL cholesterol and triglyceride levels – and this despite being high in dietary fat.

In yet another study, a low carb diet and a low fat diet were compared, the latter being compliant with the dietary guidelines of Diabetes UK. The results? The low fat diet is still inferior. Within a period of 3 months, the study's subjects lost only an average of 4.6 pounds on the low fat diet while subjects lost an average of 15.2 pounds on the low carb diet. This is one of the many dietary-fat-equals-body-fat myth busters out there.

Here's what's even better: some scientific studies on the ketogenic diet even found that it isn't necessary to count your calories in order to lose body fat on the diet. So, if you're not much of a numbers person and more of a food person, this is very good news! You can ditch the calorie counters and just focus on the right foods to eat. Personally, I find that while on the ketogenic diet, my appetite seems to naturally adjust to the point that I'm able to restrict my calories naturally as I feel full most of the time.

So how does a ketogenic diet promote healthy weight or fat loss? One of the ways by which it does so is higher intake of proteins, as a ketogenic diet inadvertently increases one's protein intake as a result of drastically cutting down or even eliminating carbohydrates.

Another reason is caloric restriction. When you eliminate or drastically cut carbs and increase fat and protein intake, you tend to feel much fuller for longer, naturally leading to less food intake. The fuller feeling is also due to significant changes in key hunger hormones such as ghrelin and leptin as a result of going on a ketogenic diet.

Other mechanisms by which a ketogenic diet helps you lose body fat are gluconeogenesis and lipogenesis. Glucogenesis is a metabolic process where fat and proteins are used as fuel by the body, which leads to an increase in daily calories burned. Lipogenesis on the other hand, is a metabolic process that converts sugar into body fat. A ketogenic diet is one that promotes glucogenesis and minimizes lipogenesis.

Lastly, a ketogenic diet is natural metabolism booster. The faster your metabolism is, the more body fat you burn on a daily basis.

Ketogenic Diet and Metabolic Diseases

Metabolic syndrome, is a cluster of conditions that include the top factors that determine your risks for heart diseases, type 2 diabetes, and obesity, which are:

- Big, fat stomach (abdominal obesity);

- Elevate blood sugar;

- High bad cholesterol (LDL) levels;

- Hypertension; and

- Low good cholesterol (HDL) levels.

Fortunately, these can be managed well or even completely wiped out with significant changes in lifestyle and diet only. And one of those diet changes is a ketogenic diet. Because a ketogenic diet is one that is insanely low in carbohydrate intake, if any, it is quite useful for bringing insulin levels down especially for people in a pre-diabetic state or with type 2 diabetes already. Insulin is produced by the body in response to increase in blood sugar, which is a direct result of the amount of carbohydrates one consumes. By reducing carbohydrate intake to practically zero, the body doesn't have to produce as much insulin, which naturally leads to lower insulin levels. Insulin levels also play a big role in obesity and significant changes in insulin levels is another mechanism by which the ketogenic diet is able to help people lose weight.

CHAPTER 3: A Ketogenic Mind

The beautiful thing about the ketogenic diet is that it comes with lots of other bonuses together with its weight loss feature. One in particular is its positive effect on the brain.

Brain-ergy

One such benefit is enhanced brain functioning, which runs contrary to many people's beliefs about the role of carbohydrates in achieving optimal mental performance. In particular, the myth states that the brain needs at least 130 grams of carbs daily for peak mental performance. This is one of the many reasons why people are very reluctant to go on an extremely low or no carb diet. Or maybe that's just an excuse to not skip on a donut or two a day – I don't know.

Nothing can be farther from the truth! According to one report published by the Food and Nutrition Board of the US Institute of Medicine, for as long as a person consumes adequate amounts of dietary fat and protein, then a person can effectively ditch carbs from his or her diet.

But this doesn't mean you should totally skip the carbs. As good as ditching carbs sound like, it's still possible to have too much of a good thing and if Brian May of the legendary band Queen wrote a song called Too Much Love Will Kill You, then you can sing another song called Too Much Carb Reduction Won't Kill You But Won't Be Optimal For Overall Health. What it is saying though is that you shouldn't worry about dropping your carbohydrate intake to just 5% of your total daily caloric consumption. At such a low level, you can still get the necessary nutrients from carbohydrate-rich sources and go keto!

So how does this happen? Diets that are very low in carbohydrates rely on 2 processes to feed the brain with enough energy: gluconeogenesis and ketogenesis. Let's explain in detail. That's why many people feel that carbs are the only way by which the brain can be energized. But while the brain can't use fat directly, it doesn't mean it can't use its derivative product. Ketogenesis is the process by which your body converts fat into ketones, which the brain can use for energy. Your liver produces ketones from fats and it does so in small amounts even when you eat normally, i.e., high carb intake. However, the production of ketones is minimal under that scenario and only increases by leaps and bounds under a state of constantly low glucose and insulin levels, which is a byproduct of consuming only 30 grams or less of carbs daily. When your carbohydrate intake's less than 50 grams or even eliminated, your brain can get as much as 70% of its energy requirements from ketones.

Take note however, that 70% is just about the maximum amount of brain-ergy (brain energy) that ketones can provide. Therefore, it still needs about 30% from carbs. That's why a little bit of carbohydrates every day is still recommended for optimal brain function. But even then, there will still be some deficit, given the less than 30 grams daily limit. Here's where gluconeogenesis comes in.

Gluconeogenesis is a process that literally means to make or create new glucose. Once again, the liver plays the primary role as it converts amino acids and glycerol into glucose.

Together, ketogenesis and glucogenesis form a dynamic duo of Batman and Robin, respectively, in helping eliminate brain fog and optimize your mental performance.

Epileptic Connection

Epilepsy affects millions of people all over the world, especially children. While there are many drugs on the market that help control, minimize or stop seizures, there's still a significant portion of those afflicted with the condition that drugs can't seem to help. When epilepsy's unresponsive to drugs, it's called a refractory kind of epilepsy.

So what's the connection with the ketogenic diet? Well for starters, its pioneer – Dr. Russell Wilder – didn't really have fat loss in mind when he created the diet. The purpose for which he created the ketogenic diet was to help children with refractory epilepsy! His original version of the ketogenic diet involved getting as much as 90% of daily calories from fat, which was found to copy the same benefits starvation brings to people who suffer from epileptic seizures.

But how does a ketogenic diet help treat refractory epilepsy? No one knows for sure as the real processes behind the effect remain unknown.

Ketogenesis and Alzheimer's disease

Based on a limited number of formal studies, the ketogenic diet appears to be helpful to people afflicted with Alzheimer's disease, which is a form of dementia that affects many people all over the world. It's a brain condition that eventually leads to loss of memory. For many scientists, Alzheimer's may be considered some kind of 3rd type of diabetes. It's with Alzheimer's, the brain is unable to properly utilize glucose as a source of energy and becomes insulin resistant, both of which result in brain inflammation. And because a ketogenic diet forces the brain to feed primarily on ketones instead of glucose for energy, it accounts for the reported beneficial effects on Alzheimer's patients.

One of the few studies done on the link between a ketogenic diet and improvements in Alzheimer's involved 152 subjects suffering from the condition. They were given a Medium Chain Triglyceride (MCT) supplement for 3 months, after which significantly higher ketone levels and remarkable improvements in mental functioning and performance were observed.

As with epilepsy, the underlying mechanism by which ketogenesis leads to improvements in Alzheimer's patients is yet to be established. But one potential explanation for the beneficial effects of ketones is protection of brain cells through the reduction of reactive oxygen species that are considered to be inflammatory byproducts of metabolism. Another potential explanation is that a high fat diet helps reduce the amount of harmful proteins that build up inside the brains of Alzheimer's patients.

Other Brain-efits Of the Ketogenic Diet

As your favorite infomercial programs often say after rattling off thousands of benefits that you can enjoy with the products they are pitching on late night TV, but wait...there's more! Some of the other benefits to the brain as a result of being in consistent state of ketosis include:

- Assists in recovery from traumatic brain injuries as high blood sugar resulting from high carbohydrate intake can stand in the way of full recover by patients;

- Beneficial effects – even successful treatment – of a condition called congenital hyperinsulinism, which can ultimately lead to brain damage;

- Improved memory, especially in Alzheimer's patients;

- Improved mental performance;

- Improvement in symptoms of Parkinson's disease; and

- Migraine relief.

CHAPTER 4: How to Go On a Ketogenic Diet

The beautiful thing about the ketogenic diet, as mentioned earlier, is that it's very practical. It's not about limiting you to eating exotic food that you can only find in some far away hidden continent each and every day but it's about letting you eat a wide variety of foods that you love and that are easily available just about anywhere. Of course, the only limitation is that it must have very low levels of carbs, i.e., less than 30 grams daily.

For a clearer idea of how to go on a ketogenic diet, here are the guidelines:

- Don't be afraid to experiment with different foods, recipes and combos until you get the keto-combo that works best for you;

- Eat low-carbohydrate veggies to help you feel fuller and take in important phytonutrients;

- Keep at it with consistency and persistence as success doesn't come overnight;

- Keep your carbs in check by reading food labels and limiting daily consumption to a maximum of 30 grams only;

- Keep your pantry stocked up with the most important food staples such as cream, oily fish, avocados, oils, nuts, eggs, cheese and meat;

- Monitor your ketogenic progress by taking before and after photos, body measurements, and weight, evaluate after 3 to 4 weeks, and if necessary, adjust your eating accordingly;

- Plan your meals and days so that you minimize the risk of being forced to eat a high carb meal, especially when dining out; and

- Supplement your diet with salt, some magnesium or electrolytes, MCT oil (up to 10 grams twice daily) and coconut oil.

Foods You Can Eat

Apart from its ability to help people lose weight, mostly body fat, the ketogenic diet is also very popular because it's actually a very delicious one, with a wide range of non-carbohydrate fare you can choose from such as:

- Avocados;
- Bacon;
- Chia Seeds;
- Chicken;

- Eggs (omega-3 or pastured);

- Grass-Fed Cream and Butter, If Possible;

- Ham;

- Healthy Oils like Avocado, Coconut, and Olive Oils;

- Low carb condiments such as herbs, spices, pepper, and salt;

- Mackerel;

- Nuts;

- Red Meat;

- Salmon;

- Sausage;

- Steak;

- Trout;

- Tuna;

- Turkey;

- Unprocessed Cheeses; and

- Vegetables with very low carb content such as peppers, onions, tomatoes, etc.

Banned Foods

These are mostly carbohydrate-rich fare such as:

- All fruits except a small amount of berries;

- Any alcoholic beverages as most of them have high carb content;

- Condiments or seasonings that are high in unhealthy fat like mayonnaise and processed vegetable oils;

- Diet or low fat food products, which are often times laden with "hidden" carbs;

- High sugar condiments like ketchup;

- High Sugar Content Stuff such as candies, cakes, ice creams, fruit juices, smoothies, etc.;

- Legumes and beans like chickpeas, lentils, kidney beans, and peas;

- Starches or grains like cereals, pastas, rice, and any wheat-based food; and

- Tubers and root veggies like parsnips, carrots, sweet potatoes, and potatoes.

Possible Issues Concerning Low-Carb and Ketogenic Diets

Nothing in this world is perfect, and that includes the ketogenic diet. For all its great benefits, here are some of the potential side effects of trying to be in a consistent state of ketosis:

- Although it seldom happens, kidney stones have been known to occur in children who used the ketogenic diet as treatment for refractory epilepsy and are usually managed using potassium citrate;

- Constipation, which can be mitigated by taking fiber supplements like psyllium fiber husks, which are practically carb-free;

- Keto flu or low-carb flu, which involves headaches, lethargy and lightheadedness for a few days only;

- Muscle cramps; and

- High cholesterol levels in both adults and children, and high triglyceride levels in children, which may only be temporary and may not necessarily affect cardiovascular health.

Ketogenic Adaptation Tips

To minimize the chances of experiencing the above-mentioned side effects, you must drink enough fluids. To be exact, drink a minimum of 2 liters or 68 ounces of water daily to replenish body fluids lost in the initial stages of ketosis. You can also increase your salt intake up to 2 extra grams daily to replace lost salts through urination due to carb depletion. Try drinking broth, which can assist you to meet both fluid and sodium needs daily. You can also take magnesium and potassium supplements or load up in foods high in both – such as fish, tomatoes, Greek yogurt, and avocados – to minimize your risks of muscle cramps.

If you're the type who's actively engaged in strenuous physical activities such as lifting weights, running or cross-fit, you might want to bring the intensity levels several notches down in the first week. Your body needs ample time to adapt to replacing carbs and glycogen with ketones as its primary fuel source for the muscles and, as such, you'll find it quite challenging to exercise with the same intensity as you normally do within the first week or two. So, don't push it until your body's fully adapted to ketosis.

CHAPTER 5: Ketogenic Myths and Old Wives' Tales

Just like with your favorite celebrities, there are many rumors, myths and old wives' tales circulating concerning the ketogenic diet – particularly evil ones! In this chapter, I shall attempt to debunk those malicious claims against the ketogenic diet and shall play the role of a ketogenic apologetic (translated as defender of the ketogenic faith)! Here are some of the most common misconceptions about living la vida low-carb!

Low Means No

For some strange reason, many well-meaning and highly educated people can't tell the difference between the 2 words, particularly as applied to low carbohydrates and no carbohydrates, and assume that both are the same. Nothing can be farther from the truth! God made your body in such a way that it needs carbohydrates to function optimally – the only thing that's up for debate is how much of it should comprise your daily caloric intake! In fact, without carbs, your body may not be able to perform key metabolic functions like glycol-protein and mucus production, as well as the maintenance of your cells' integrity. Going no carb can even increase your cortisol (stress hormone) levels and reduce testosterone levels.

That's why, if you remember from earlier, we pegged the limit at 30 grams daily, which is a good enough consumption that strikes a good balance between giving your body enough carbs to function normally while losing body fat and staying healthy and energetic.

The Paleo-Genic Diet

Another popular misconception about the ketogenic is that one is Superman and the other is Clark Kent – they're both one and the same! While the Paleo diet can be ketogenic in the sense that it can also be high fat and low carb, it can be just the opposite, i.e., high carb and low fat. Why? It's because the basis of all things paleo isn't in the carbs-to-fat ratio but in the types of food you eat. Basically, the Paleo diet's all about eating food that primitive people or Neanderthals ate long, long ago, which can be high-fat-low-carb or high-carb-low-fat, depending on what's available.

Plants versus Keto

Another popular misconception about the ketogenic diet is that you shouldn't eat veggies while on the diet because it's "carbs" and as such, you can miss out on important nutrients. Again, we'll have to go back to the Low Means No myth to see the reason behind this rumor.

The ketogenic diet doesn't necessarily ban all kinds of fruits and veggies. In fact, go back to the list of allowed foods in Chapter 4 and you'll see that low carbohydrate veggies – like broccoli, cabbage, and lettuce – are in the list as well as berries and avocadoes – in the right amounts of course. What's banned – if you want to use the word – in the ketogenic diet are very starchy vegetables and high sugar fruits due to their very high carbohydrate content.

The Atkins Diet Reincarnation

The Atkins diet has been around like, you know – forever – and that makes it one of the most popular low carb diets around. And the "low" or "no" carbs portion is the main reason the ketogenic diet's been accused of being the reincarnation or pirated copy of the Atkins diet.

With all due respect to the late Dr. Atkins, his diet's totally different from the ketogenic diet because of its high protein – often times it becomes excess protein – mantra. Too much protein can still raise insulin levels and increase your risk for obesity because of a familiar process called – wait for it – gluconeogenesis! If you recall, it's a process by which the liver produces carbohydrates from proteins. So, if you go on the Atkins diet thinking it's basically the same as going keto like Clark Kent ditches his glasses and clothes to become Superman, you'll fail to achieve nutritional ketosis due to excess protein.

Excess Red Meat Is Nutritionally Evil

The myth here is not in the fact that it really is – nutritionally speaking – evil to consume too much red meat but in the belief that going ketogenic automatically translates to excess consumption of red meat! No, it doesn't because remember, red meat isn't the only food you get to eat on the diet – there are many others like poultry, fish, and oils which make it highly unlikely to overload on red meat on a daily basis unless you intentionally do so. But think about it, you can overload on red meats on any diet you choose to do whether it's the Atkins Diet, the Paleo Diet, or the See Food (when you see food, you eat) diet! No diet has the exclusive claim to excess consumption of red meats! Oh, and it's not only red meat where excess consumption is nutritionally bad – the same goes for just about everything else, including water!

CHAPTER 6: Easy Ketogenic Recipes

Ok...here's where the rubber – pardon the pun – meats the road! Here are a couple of recipes to help you start your ketogenic journey in a practically delicious note! They're not only delish but are quite easy to prepare too, with no exotic ingredients necessary.

Bon appetite!

For Breakfast

Benedictine Eggs

Ingredients:

- 4 Bacon Strips; and

- 4 Whole Eggs.

Instructions:

- Bring your oven to 350 degrees Fahrenheit and while doing so, line a muffin baking sheets cups with bacon strips.

- After breaking the eggs, pour the contents in the bacon-lined muffin cups and bake for about 10 minutes or until your desired consistency is achieved.

- Enjoy with parsley garnishes.

Kevlar Coffee (Bulletproof)

Ingredients:

- 2 Cups Coffee (Ground);
- 2 Tablespoons of Virgin Coconut Oil;
- 2 Tablespoons of Grass-Fed Butter (Unsalted);

Instructions:

- After brewing your favorite ground coffee per your preference, drop the unsalted butter in it and let the butter melt fully before doing the same with the coconut oil.
- Mix very well and enjoy!

For Lunch

Crispy Choppers

Ingredients:

- 1 Tablespoon of Grass-Fed Butter;
- 1 Teaspoon of Black Pepper;
- 1 Teaspoon of Salt;
- ½ Cup of Flour (Coconut);
- ¼ Teaspoon of Cayenne Pepper; and
- 3 Pieces of Pork Chops.

Instructions:

- In a medium-sized container with a lid, combine all the dry ingredients for the coating for the pork chops.
- Put the pork chops in the container and cover with the lid. Shake to evenly coat the chops.
- In a medium-sized skillet set over medium-high heat, melt the butter. Cook the coated pork chops in the butter for up to 5 minutes per side or until the pork chops aren't pink anymore.

This Is Not Mr. Bean's Chili

Ingredients:

- 1 ½ Teaspoons of Cumin;
- 1 Cup of Broth (Beef);
- 1 Medium-Sized Green Pepper;
- 1 Medium-Sized Onion;
- 1 Teaspoon + 2 Tablespoons of Chili Powder;
- 1 Teaspoon of Black Pepper;
- 1 Teaspoon of Cayenne Pepper;
- 1 Teaspoon of Oregano;
- 1 Teaspoon of Salt;
- 1 Teaspoon of Worcestershire Sauce;
- 1/3 Cup of Tomato Paste;
- 2 Pounds of Ground Chicken or Beef;
- 2 Tablespoons of Olive Oil;
- 2 Tablespoons of Soy Sauce;
- 2 Teaspoons of Minced Garlic; and
- 2 Teaspoons of Smoked Paprika

Instructions:

- Prepare your slow cooker.
- Sautee the ground chicken or beef in a big-sized skillet until cooked through. When done, transfer the sautéed ground chicken or beef into the slow cooker.
- Combine all of the spices, oil, tomato paste, and Worcestershire sauce in a mixing bowl before pouring the mixture in the slow cooker to marinate the ground meat.
- Meanwhile, chop the onion and green pepper and sauté them in the skillet with the remaining fat from the meat you sautéed earlier. Cook until the onions turn translucent and brown. Pour the sautéed veggies – including the fat in which they were cooked – in the slow cooker. Stir well before covering the cooker.
- Set the cooker on high setting and cook the chili for 2 ½ hours. Remove the cover at the

2-hour mark to allow the chili to simmer for the remaining 30 minutes.

- You can add jalapeno peppers if you'd like a strong spice kick.

For Dinner

Omega Seafood Salad

Ingredients:

- 1 Can Of Tuna Packed In Water;
- 1 Cooked Egg, Chopped;
- 1 Small White Onion, Chopped;
- 1 Tablespoon of Mayonnaise;
- 1 Tablespoon of Sour Cream;
- 1/8 Teaspoon of Cayenne Pepper;
- ¼ Cup of Monterey Jack Cheese, Shredded;
- ¼ Teaspoon of Dill;
- 2 Bacon Slices;
- Lettuce or Cabbage; and
- 2 Teaspoons of Dijon Mustard

Instructions:

- In a skillet set on medium-high heat, melt the butter and cook the bacon strips in it until they turn brown and crispy.
- In a mixing bowl, mix together well the herbs and spices, sour cream, and mayonnaise. Mix the cheese, chopped egg and diced onions in and mix thoroughly.
- Crumble the bacon strips and mix it into the tuna mixture before serving over a bed of lettuce or cabbage.

Coco Loco Soup with Shrimps

Ingredients:

- 1 Lime's Worth Of Juice;

- 1 Onion, Diced;

- 1 Pound of Shrimps, Already Peeled;

- 1 Red Bell Pepper, Diced;

- 2 Cans of Coconut Milk, Unsweetened;

- 2 Cloves of Garlic, Minced;

- 2 Cups of Veggie Stock;

- 2 Tablespoons of Cilantro;

- 2 Tablespoons of Grass-Fed Butter; and

- 2 Tablespoons of Red Curry Paste

Instructions:

- In a big-sized pot set on medium-high heat, melt the butter and cook the shrimps in it for up to 3 minutes or until pink. While cooking, season with pepper and salt for taste and set aside in another container when done.

- In the same pot, throw in the bell pepper, onion, and garlic and cook for up to 4 minutes or until veggies turn tender.

- Mix in the ginger and cook for another minute or until fragrant. Mix the curry paste in before gradually adding the veggie stock and coconut milk in the pot. Continue whisking until thoroughly combined.

- Allow the mixture to come to a boil before reducing the heat. Allow simmering for up to 10 minutes or until thick.

- Add the shrimps back in together with the lime juice and enjoy with cilantro garnishing.

CHAPTER 7: How to Stay On the Ketogenic Path When Eating Out

Whether it's the ketogenic diet or some other diet, one of the biggest challenges when it comes to staying the course is eating out. Given that the ketogenic diet isn't as restrictive as other diets, that challenge can be easily overcome by doing the following.

Include Fat – The Healthy Kind

Because of the common misconception that dietary fat is the child of the devil when it comes to health and fitness, many restaurants want to look all goody two shoes by offering many meals that are low in it. However, that makes it hard for carb-less meals to be very satisfying. Fortunately, there's something you can do about that: just ask for extra butter and put it on your meat and veggies to melt and mix. For salads (how low fat can you get, eh?), you can simply ask for dressing made from vinegar and olive oil and drizzle your salad generously with it to add healthy dietary fat to your low fat fare.

However, keep in mind that most restaurants – especially the low end commercial ones – don't keep stock of olive oil but instead, use cheaper versions of vegetable oil that are significantly less healthy. You can do what many other seasoned ketogenic dieters do – bring your own small bottle of olive oil.

Go Starchless

Ignore the rice, potatoes, pasta and bread when eating out. To help you resist the temptation, tell the person taking your order to serve your ordered meal without the starchy carbs that usually come along with them. In most restaurants, entrees would usually be served with a replacement salad or additional vegetables in lieu of the starchy carbs you want to remove. If the restaurant doesn't replace your ditched carbs – don't worry. Just order your dish sans the starchy carbs and order a leafy veggie side dish that's very low in carbs to go with it. Don't tempt yourself by letting your orders be served together with the usual starchy carbs that come with them believing your will power's as strong as Dwayne "The Rock" Johnson's muscles. You might be disappointed to find that it's only as strong as Peewee Herman's when it comes to resisting those deliciously tempting starchy carb sides.

Reflect On Your Desserts

If you're at a crossroads as to whether or not you'll enjoy dessert, ask yourself: am I – after all that fat and protein – still hungry? Chances are that you're not hungry anymore and it's more likely your sweet tooth that's trying to call the shots. If so, a good compromise would be to just go for a good cup of tea or coffee (if already evening, maybe decaf) with a good and healthy sugar substitute like stevia for a nice sweet but carb-less taste.

Watch the Condiments and Sauces

Many condiments or sauces – such as Béarnaise sauce – have very little content other than fat while others – such as ketchups – lie on the other end of the spectrum, with no other calories except for carbohydrates. It's the same with gravies, which can be both!

Just to be sure, ask the chef or waiter what a particular sauce is made of. Keep particular attention if he or she says it contains flour or sugar. And if you really can't help it, just ask for the sauce to be segregated on the side so that you can control how much of it you'll eat with your meal.

Conclusion

There you have it – the ketogenic diet. Now that you've finished reading this book and have learned what the ketogenic diet's all about, it's benefits, it's potential side-effects (and how to minimize them), how to go on a ketogenic diet, a couple of deliciously practical recipes to help you hit the ground running, and how to stay keto while eating out, you're in a great position to start losing weight.

However, knowing is just half the battle – the other half is action or application of knowledge. As such, you must start applying what you learned a.s.a.p. Because the longer you put it off, the higher your risk becomes of not starting at all. And if you don't, you won't lose the excess body fat you want to lose. So act now.

Thank you again for buying this book. And if you enjoyed this book, then I'd like to ask you for a favor, would you be kind enough to leave a review for this book on Amazon? It'd be greatly appreciated!

Click here to leave a review for this book on Amazon!

Thank you and good luck!

Printed in Great Britain
by Amazon